Back Pain

Natural Drug Free Remedies to Cure Chronic Back Pain Permanently

Robert S. Lee

Contents

Chapter 1. Back Pain & Some Common Causes

There are many people who suffer from back pain, but that doesn't mean you have to put up with it or turn to over the counter medication or prescription drugs to treat it. There are natural options and alternatives to you, which will help you to get your back pain under control and reduce your risk of flare-ups even when suffering from chronic pain. Anyone can suffer from back pain. It doesn't matter how old you are or what walk of life you come from. Sadly, back pain actually becomes more common as you age, and many people first get back pain between the ages of thirty to forty years old.

Common Causes for Back Pain:

If you have poor physical fitness, then you're much more likely to suffer from back pain than those who are fit. Another factor that puts you at a higher risk for back pain is being overweight, which is why maintaining a healthy weight can help you to manage back pain if you already have it. This is because too much weight puts stress on your back, which can cause chronic back pain.

Sadly, there are people who are predisposed to back pain just because of their genetics. Especially if arthritis runs in your family, and there are some types of arthritis that does affect the spine. If you have a job that strains your back, you're more likely to experience back pain as well. Bad posture can also result in reoccurring pain, as well as smoking. This is because if you smoke your body is less likely to provide the disks in your back with the nutrients it needs.

Knowing When to Treat:

You should never let your back pain get out of hand, which is why it's important to know when to start treating back pain. If you are experiencing back pain that doesn't get better with rest, then you know that you have a problem, and should start looking into treatment methods. Numbness and tingling are also a severe symptom of chronic back pain that tells you that you've let it go on too long.

If you are experiencing weakness or strain in your back, then you know that you should treat your back pain as well. Even minor back pain can be treated through natural means safely. If your back pain is interfering with your life, no matter if it's social, work, or school related, then you need to treat it. You should also make sure that it doesn't affect your sleep. There is no reason to deal with back pain, as there are herbal and natural solutions.

Chapter 2. Teas to Help with Chronic Back Pain

A warm tea is sure to help you melt your tension away, which is one cause of back pain. Of course, with the right tea you'll find that they are specially blended to target your back pain and get rid of it quickly. These teas are easy to make, and most of them are meant to be drank warm. However, some people will chill them before drinking.

Tea #1 Pain Relieving Blend

This is an inflammation reducing blend, and it'll help to decrease your back pain almost immediately. Inflammation can be the leading cause of back pain, and it can even cause chronic back pain. Drinking this tea once daily can help, but you can drink it two to three times daily if necessary. Ginger and turmeric are a great way to deal with inflammation.

Ingredients:

1. 2 Tablespoons Ginger, Grated

2. 1 Teaspoon Turmeric Powder

3. 1 Cup Water

4. 2 Teaspoons Honey, Raw

Directions:

1. Boil your water, and then put in your ginger and turmeric powder. Make sure that you let it steep for seven to nine minutes.

2. Strain out the herbs and add in the honey. Stir until completely dissolved, and it's recommended you drink this tea warm.

Tea #2 Lemongrass & Ginger

You already know that ginger is a great way to relieve inflammation, but when you add it to lemongrass you have a potent combination to help you relieve your back pain quickly. Lemongrass is known as a natural pain killer, and one of the best parts is that you can grow it easily in a container right in your backyard or even in your home. Fresh lemongrass is always best, but dried lemongrass will work if you're in a pinch.

Ingredients:

1. 1 Tablespoon Ginger, Grated

2. 2 Tablespoons Lemon Grass, Fresh

3. 2 Teaspoons Honey, Raw

4. 1 Cup Water

Direction:

1. Boil the cup of water, adding in your lemongrass and ginger. Take it off heat and let it steep for eight to ten minutes.

2. Strain out the herbs, and add in your honey, stirring until fully dissolved. Drink while warm.

Tea #3 Chamomile Tea

What many people don't realize is that back pain can be caused by tension, which is made worse by anxiety and stress. Chamomile can help with all three, so sometimes a chamomile tea is all you need to help get rid of your back pain. Keeping your stress away is important, and dried chamomile can be found in most any local grocery store.

Ingredients:

1. 2 Tablespoons Chamomile Flowers, Dried

2. 1 ½ Teaspoons Honey, Raw

3. 1 Cup Water

Directions:

1. Boil the water, and then take it off heat. Add in your chamomile flowers, and then let steep for six to eight minutes.

2. Strain out the chamomile flowers, and then add in the honey. Stir until it's dissolved and then drink while still warm.

Tea #4 Ginger & Spice

Cayenne pepper is known to help relieve back pain, and ginger is a great inflammation relief as well. With a little added spice you'll find that this will not only kick your pain, but it'll also kick your metabolism into gear. It can help with joint pain as well. Cinnamon is known to help you with muscle pain, and it adds in well to this spiced ginger tea to help relieve your back pain quickly. You can drink it throughout the day as necessary.

Ingredients:

1. 1 Cup Water

2. ½ Teaspoon Cayenne Pepper Powder

3. 2 Tablespoons Ginger, Grated

4. ½ Teaspoon Cinnamon, Ground

5. 2 Teaspoons Honey, Raw

Directions:

1. Boil your cup of water, adding in all other ingredients except for honey. Let steep after taking off heat for six to eight minutes.

2. Strain out all herbs, and then add in your honey. Drink while warm.

Tea #5 Cinnamon & Fennel

You already know that cinnamon can help you with pain relief in your muscles, but fennel can as well. It provides a licorice flavored tea that is sure to relieve your pain quickly. It's great for cramping, which will help your tension to be relieved quickly. It can even help with chronic back pain.

Ingredients:

1. 1 Teaspoon Fennel Seeds, Crushed

2. 1 Cup Water

3. 1 Teaspoon Cinnamon, Ground

4. 1 ½ Teaspoon Honey, Raw

Directions:

1. Boil the cup of water, and then add in your crushed fennel seeds and cinnamon. Take it off heat, letting steep for six to eight minutes.

2. Strain, and then add honey to drink while warm.

Tea #6 White Willow Bark

White willow bark is a great way to relieve pain, and it's been sued for centuries. Just remember to sweeten with honey, and you don't need to add anything else. Remember that you can't take willow bark if you are allergic to aspirin.

Ingredients:

1. 2 Teaspoons White Willow Bark

2. 1 Cup Water

3. 1 Teaspoon Honey, Raw

Directions:

1. Boil the water, and then take it off heat. Add in the white willow bark, and let it steep for fifteen to twenty minutes.

2. Strain out the white willow bark and add in your honey, making sure it's

thoroughly dissolved before drinking. You can reheat if necessary.

Tea #7 Peppermint & Lemongrass

You already know that lemongrass is a pain reliever in general, but peppermint is actually going to help relieve your back pain specifically. The menthol and camphor are great at relieving back pain, and they help to ease the tightness in your muscles.

Ingredients:

1. 2 Tablespoons Peppermint Leaves, Dried

2. 1 Tablespoon Lemongrass, Fresh

3. 1 Teaspoon Honey, Raw

4. 1 Cup Water

Directions:

1. Boil the water, and then take off heat, adding in the lemongrass and peppermint leaves.

2. Let steep for eight to ten minutes, and then strain the herbs out.

3. Stir in honey, and drink while warm.

Chapter 3. Salves That Will Do the Trick Fast

Having a salve to rub onto your back will help you to make sure that you can get rid of your back pain fast. Sometimes you don't have the time for a tea to kick in, and you don't want to wait for medicine to kick in either, even herbal supplements. This is where salves come in, and they can be stored for a long time and made in advance. They're even easy to take with you if you need instant relief.

Salve #1 Cayenne Heating Salve

If you're looking for a heating salve, then you'll find that cayenne will do the trick. Cayenne is known to help with pain when applied internally and externally, and that's why it can be used in a salve as well as a tea, but you'll find that when applied directly to the muscles, it will work quicker and more effectively. The heat will help to relax your muscles quickly, which can provide nearly instant pain relief in your back. Remember to wash your hands after applying and do not get around your nose, eyes or mouth or you will experience burning.

Ingredients:

1. ½ Cup Olive Oil, Extra Virgin

2. ½ Ounce Beeswax, Grated

3. 2 Teaspoons Cayenne Powder

Directions:

1. Take a double boiler and put together your olive oil and your beeswax together. Turn it over low heat, and melt together, stirring so it doesn't burn and combines.

2. Once melted and combined, add in the cayenne powder, making sure it is mixed evenly. Take off heat.

3. Pour into prepared containers. A glass jar or airtight tin is usually best. Apply to the area as needed.

Salve #2 Cooling Salve

This is a cooling salve, and if you can't handle the heat of the cayenne pepper salve, then you'll find that this salve can help your back pain as well. It's cool and refreshing, and it'll help with even chronic pain. Make sure that you apply it whenever you feel the start of pain for the best results. Eucalyptus oil will help to relieve tension, as well as camphor oil and peppermint oil.

Ingredients:

1. ½ Cup Coconut Oil

2. 2 Teaspoon Beeswax, Grated

3. 5-6 Drops Camphor Oil

4. 5-6 Drops Peppermint Essential Oil

5. 5 Drops Eucalyptus Essential Oil

Directions:

1. Take a double boiler putting it on low heat, and then add in your beeswax and your coconut oil. Make sure it melts together, stirring so it does not burn and combines evenly.

2. Take off heat, stirring in your oils, making sure it's blended well before pouring it into containers to firm and cool before sealing. Apply to the affected area as needed.

Salve #3 Comfrey Cooling Salve

Comfrey leaves are a great way of helping to make sure that you relieve your back pain quickly. It can help with back pain, bruises, sprains, and even arthritis. It is an all over pain relieving salve that will help you to experience relief quickly. With peppermint added in it has a cooling effect that helps to relax the muscles, helping you to get relief even faster.

Ingredients:

1. 10 Drops Peppermint Essential Oil

2. ½ Cup Coconut Oil

3. 2 Teaspoons Beeswax, Grated

4. ¼ Cup Comfrey Leaves, Dried

Directions:

1. Take the comfrey leaves and add them to the coconut oil, putting both in a medium

saucepan and simmering over low heat for one hour to infuse the oil. Make sure to stir periodically to keep it from burning, and then strain out the comfrey leaves.

2. Place a double boiler over low heat, and add in the infused oil and beeswax. Mix together until blended, and then blend in the peppermint essential oil.

3. Take off heat, and pour into prepared containers to cool and firm before sealing. Apply when you start to feel pain.

Salve #4 Blended Arnica Salve

Arnica flowers are also known to help with back pain. They're a strong herb for topical pain relief, and you'll find that lavender will help you to make sure that your stress isn't causing tension. The peppermint also relaxes muscles and relieves the tension that could be causing your back pain. You'll relieve muscle tension and reduce inflammation with this wonderful arnica blended salve.

Ingredients:

1.   ¼ Teaspoon Lavender Essential oil

2. ¼ Teaspoon Peppermint Essential Oil

3. ½ Cup Beeswax Granules

4. 6 Ounces Arnica Flowers, Dried

5. 2 Cups Coconut Oil

Directions:

1. Place the coconut oil in a large saucepan over low heat for one hour with the arnica flowers in it. Stir in, and continue to stir occasionally to keep it from burning. Afterwards, strain out the flowers and keep the arnica infused coconut oil.

2. Take a double boiler over low heat, and then melt the coconut oil and beeswax together to combine. Add in essential oils, and then pour into prepared containers to firm and cool before applying to the area and storing.

Salve #5 Plantain Salve

Most people consider plantain to be a weed, but it can be an extremely helpful herb to have for a pain relieving salve. It can help to relieve back pain topically be decreasing inflammation. Plantain is even great for rashes and bruises. The peppermint oil adds a soothing effect, and clove oil is known to be a topical numbing agent, which will help to speed the pain relief along.

Ingredients:

1. 2 Teaspoons Beeswax, Grated

2. ½ Cup Coconut Oil

3. 10 Drops Peppermint Essential Oil

4. 5 Drops Clove Essential Oil

5. ¼ Cup Plantain Leaves

6. 1 Teaspoon Cayenne Pepper Powder

Directions:

1. Take your coconut oil and mix in the cayenne pepper and plantain leaves. Simmer in a saucepan over low heat to infuse for two to three hours, stirring periodically so it doesn't burn.

2. Strain out the herbs, and then put in a double boiler with beeswax to melt. Mix in essential oils, and then pour into prepared containers to cool and firm before sealing.

Salve #6 Soothing Pain Relief

Lavender essential oil is known for its pain reliving properties, and this can be said for roman chamomile essential oil as well. It's anti-inflammatory and helps to relieve muscle tension, anxiety, and stress. This salve doesn't burn at all, and you can apply it as much as you need to.

Ingredients:

1. ½ Cup Coconut Oil

2. 10 Drops Peppermint Essential Oil

3. 2 Teaspoons Beeswax, Grated

4. 10 Drops Roman Chamomile Essential Oil

5. 15 Drops Lavender Essential Oil

Directions:

1. Take a double boiler and put it over low heat, combining the beeswax and coconut

oil, melting until combined. Stir so it does not burn, and then take it off heat.

2. Add in all essential oils, making sure they're mixed all the way through, and pour it into prepared airtight containers. Do not seal until cooled and firm. Apply regularly to the area as needed.

Chapter 4. Body Butter That You Can Keep for Relief

If you're suffering from back pain, you sometimes just want an all-natural lotion that you can apply a little more often, and usually with a better scent. That's what these natural body butter recipes are for. They apply more directly to the entire back, and you can use them on other muscles for pain relief as well. Each one is meant to be used like lotion, and it has a much thinner consistency than salves. However, they are often considered less potent, and should not be used for acute back pain relief.

Body Butter #1 Lavender

Lavender body butter is easy to make, and it smells great too. Lavender is known to help ease away stress, tension, and anxiety. Chronic back pain is commonly caused by the tensing of muscles due to outside factors in your life, such as stress. Lavender body butter will help you to relax these muscles and help to get rid of your back pain naturally.

Ingredients:

1. ½ Cup Shea Butter

2. ½ Cup Mango Butter

3. ½ Cup Coconut Oil

4. 1 Cup Lavender Flowers, Dried

Directions:

1. Take a blender, and blend your lavender flowers on high until they are finer.

2. Put your coconut oil in a large saucepan over low heat, and add in your lavender flowers, making sure they are stirred in well. Let steep over low heat for three to four hours, and then strain out the flowers. Remember that you have to keep stirring periodically if you don't want it to burn.

3. Take a double boiler, mixing all butters and oil together, combining. Remember that you need to stir constantly over low heat if you don't want your shea butter to become gritty.

4. Let cool in the fridge, and then take it out and whip it. Place in prepared airtight containers. Apply as desired.

Body Butter #2 Whipped Magnesium & Chamomile

If you have enough magnesium, you are less likely to experience chronic back pain, and it can help to soothe pain when you already have it. Roman chamomile flowers will also help to soothe back pain due to its anti-inflammatory effects. You'll find that after infusing your oil, this light and fluffy body butter smells great and is easy to apply. You can apply it like lotion as many times as you want per day.

Ingredients:

1. 1 Cup Shea Butter

2. ¼ Cup Coconut Oil

3. ¼ Cup Magnesium

4. ½ Cup Chamomile Flowers, Dried

Directions:

1. Take your coconut oil and put it in a large saucepan, infusing your chamomile

flowers into it by cooking on low heat for two to three hours while stirring periodically.

2. Strain out the chamomile flowers, and add all ingredients together in a double boiler, melting gently over low heat while stirring to combine.

3. Let cool in the fridge for an hour after pouring into a bowl, and then take it out and whip it until light and fluffy. Spoon into airtight containers.

Body Butter #3 Lavender & Peppermint

Lavender is already proven to help you with your back pain, but peppermint leaves are also a great addition to a body butter made from lavender. It will provide a cooling sensation which will relieve both inflammation and tension. Of course, you'll be relieving your stress at the same time. Infuse the coconut oil for longer if you want a stronger effect.

Ingredients:

1. ½ Cup Lavender Flowers, Fresh

2. ¼ Cup Peppermint Leaves, Fresh

3. ½ Cup Coconut Oil

4. 1 Cup Shea Butter

Directions:

1. Take a large saucepan, and let the lavender and peppermint infuse into your coconut oil by cooking on low heat for three to four hours. Make sure to stir periodically so that nothing sticks, and

then you can strain out the herbs, keeping the infused oil.

2. Add the infused oil to the shea butter in a double boiler, melting over low heat until combined.

3. Place in a large bowl, whip it once and it put it in the fridge to cool.

4. Once cool, take it out and then whip until light and fluffy. Spoon it into airtight containers.

Body Butter #4 Ginger & Thyme

If you're looking for a little more of an earthy body butter that doesn't smell as sweet, then look no further. This is a body butter that will help you to decrease your back pain while still helping to make sure that all inflammation is taken care of to help with chronic pain. You can apply it as a lotion to help before pain gets bad, but it is not as strong of a pain reliever as other body butters.

Ingredients:

1. ½ Cup Thyme, Fresh

2. 4 Tablespoons Ginger, Grated

3. ½ Cup Coconut Oil

4. ½ Cup Shea Butter

5. ½ Cup Cocoa Butter

Directions:

1. Take your coconut oil, putting it over low heat in a large saucepan and combining your thyme and ginger together in it. Simmer over low for four to five hours, letting it infuse as you stir periodically to keep from burning the oil.

2. Strain out all of the herbs, keeping the infused oil. Put the infused oil in the double boiler over low heat.

3. Add in your shea butter and cocoa butter, stirring periodically until combined.

4. Pour into a bowl, and then whip. Place in the fridge to cool for two hours.

5. Take out of the fridge, and then whip until light and fluffy, spooning into airtight containers for storage.

Body Butter #5 Sandalwood & Lavender

This is a body butter that has a relaxing and delightful sense that will help your back pain, but it is also known to help to calm your nerves and mind. It will help to relieve stress and anxiety, especially if used on a regular basis, which can also help to keep back pain away. Of course, sandalwood essential oil is great to reduce tension and spasming. It also helps to reduce nerve pain, which can sometimes contribute or be the cause of even chronic back pain.

Ingredients:

1. ½ Cup Lavender Flowers

2. 20 Drops Sandalwood Essential Oil

3. ½ Cup Coconut Oil

4. 1 Cup Shea Butter

Directions:

1. Take a large saucepan, combining your coconut oil and lavender flowers. Simmer over low heat, stirring periodically, for three to four hours to infuse. Strain out the flowers, and keep the infused oil, placing it in a double boiler.

2. Add in your shea butter, and melt over low heat, stirring so your shea butter does not become gritty.

3. Take off heat, pouring into a medium bowl. Add your sandalwood essential oil, making sure to combine well. Whip before placing in the fridge to cool.

4. After two hours, take it back out, and whip until light and fluffy. You can now spoon the mixture into airtight containers for later use.

Chapter 5. Bath Soaks That Help Relax Your Back

Bath soaks, commonly called bath salts, are a great way to help your back pain. A hot bath is going to naturally relax your muscles, but when you add in herbal remedies to help you decrease your back pain, it's even better. Remember to soak for thirty to forty minutes in warm water for the best results, and you can use this during the day or at night before you go to bed. Remember that some ingredients will relax you more than others, so many people prefer to take a back pain relieving bath right before bed. It will also help to promote quality sleep, helping to relieve the tension in all of your muscles so you can wake up refreshed.

Bath Soak #1 Tension Relaxing Salts

Dead sea salt is great for your skin, and Epsom salts will help to relax your muscles. You'll find that the essential oils you are using are good for stress, anxiety, muscle tension, and even spasms. It's even going to help with inflammation, and when blended together, you have a bath soak that is sure to keep your back feeling great.

Ingredients:

1. ¼ Teaspoon Roman Chamomile Essential Oil

2. 3 Tablespoons Chamomile Flowers, Dried

3. ½ Teaspoon Lavender Essential Oil

4. 4 Tablespoons Lavender Buds, Dried

5. 1 Cup Dead Sea Salt

6. 1 Cup Epsom Salts

7. 3 Tablespoons Sea Salt, Coarse

Directions:

1. Take your sea salt, mixing in your essential oils into it, and blend in a blender until smooth.

2. Stir all salts together in a large bowl, and add in dried lavender buds and

chamomile flowers until blended evenly throughout.

3. Place in an airtight container for storage, and use a ¼ cup to a ½ cup for each bath.

Bath Soak #2 Ginger & Epsom Salts

Ginger is anti-inflammatory, and this is a great bath salt if you have only mild back pain. It isn't strong in scent, but you'll find that it works on any and all of your muscles when mixed with the tension relieving properties of Epsom salts. The peppermint is what gives this bath soak its scent, and it'll also help to sooth your muscles and lighten your mood. Decreasing your stress is a great way to help decrease chronic pain.

Ingredients:

1. 6 Tablespoons Ginger, Ground

2. 10 Drops Peppermint Essential Oil

3. 1 Cup Epsom Salts

Directions:

1. Blend everything together, and then store in an airtight container until you're ready to use. Use a ¼ cup to a half cup with each bath.

Bath Soak #3 Inflammation Reliever

If you're looking for a bath soak that will help you to relieve any inflamed muscles in your back a little quicker, then you're going to want this bath soak recipe. Frankincense essential oil is known for its anti-inflammatory properties, and it's known as a general pain relieving essential oil. When combined with turmeric and ginger it provides a powerful pain relieving punch.

Ingredients:

1. 4 Tablespoons Ginger, Ground

2. 1 Tablespoon Turmeric, Ground

3. 1 Cup Epsom Salts

4. 20 Drops Frankincense Essential Oil

Directions:

1. Take a teaspoon of your Epsom salts, and then blend the essential oil into it in a blender, adding in ginger and turmeric powder.

2. Mix the blended mixture into the remaining Epsom salts. Store in an airtight container, adding a ¼ cup to a ½ cup to each bath.

Soak #4 Stress & Spasm Reducer

Stress can contribute to back pain, including chronic back pain, so reducing your stress while stopping any spasming so that your back can heal is very important. The lavender helps to reduce the stress, but sandalwood essential oil is great to keep spasms at bay. This will help to keep your muscles from tensing. Chamomile flowers top off the mixture by relaxing you so that your muscles won't spasm as well. It'll even help to relieve anxiety.

Ingredients:

1. 1 Cup Epsom Salts

2. ½ Cup Dried Lavender Flowers, Dried

3. 15 Drops Sandalwood Essential Oil

4. ¼ Cup Chamomile Flowers, Dried

Directions:

1. Blend your chamomile flowers and sandalwood essential oil together with a teaspoon of the Epsom salts in a blender.

2. Mix into the remaining Epsom salts, and mix in lavender flowers. Use ¼ to a ½ cup with each bath. Remember to soak for at least thirty minutes.

Soak #5 Nerve Pain Relief

Nerve pain is a little harder to cure when it has to do with your back, but you'll find that this back soak can really help. Juniper essential oil is great at targeting nerve pain. It also helps to relieve muscle aches and keep spasming at bay, just like the sandalwood oil. The thyme is known to relieve stress as well as relieve general backache.

Ingredients:

1. 20 Drops Juniper Essential Oil

2. 10-15 Drops Sandalwood Essential Oil

3. 1 Cup Epsom Salts

4. 2 Tablespoons Thyme, Dried

Directions:

1. Blend all ingredients together. Blend your thyme in a blender to make smaller if necessary first. Make sure that your essential oils do not clump up when

mixing throughout the Epsom salts. Use
¼ to a ½ cup depending on the severity
of pain with each bath.

2.

Bath Soak #6 Earthy Pain Relief

The smell of lemon is known to help uplift your
spirits, which many people who experience back
pain could use. Thyme is known to help relieve
general muscle pain, especially back pain. The
real addition to this bath soak mix is the
rosemary, which is able to relieve both joint and
muscle pain, helping your back in multiple ways.

Ingredients:

1. 2 Tablespoons Lemon Zest

2. 3 Tablespoons Thyme, Dried

3. ¼ Cup Rosemary, Dried

4. 1 Cup Epsom Salts

Directions:

1. Take a tablespoon of your Epsom salts, adding your rosemary, lemon zest, and thyme into a blender with it. Blend until smaller.

2. Mix everything together and store in an airtight container. Depending on the severity of your pain and mood, add ¼ to a ½ cup with each bath.

Bath Soak #7 Chamomile & Peppermint

This is a simple bath soak recipe for mild back pain. It targets stress, tension, general muscle pain, and even inflammation. You won't smell the ginger under the peppermint and chamomile, but it takes care of any mild inflammation that may be adding to your back pain.

Ingredients:

1. 20-25 Drops Peppermint Essential Oil

2. ½ Cup Chamomile Flowers

3. 1 Teaspoon Ginger, Dried

4. 1 Cup Epsom Salts

Directions:

1. Blend a tablespoon of your Epsom salts with your essential oil in a blender until smooth.

2. Add the mixture to the rest of your Epsom salts, mixing all ingredients together before storing in an airtight container.

Bath Soak #8 Lemongrass Pain Relief

This is an overall pain reliever, which is helpful for back pain as well. Lemongrass is the main star of this back pain remedy, as the essential oil is known to be an overall pain reliever. However, wintergreen essential oil helps it along for the same reason, helping it to pack powerful pain relieving properties.

Ingredients:

1. 10 Drops Lemongrass Essential Oil

2. 10 Drops Wintergreen Essential Oil

3. 4 Tablespoons Lemongrass, Dried

4. 1 Cup Epsom Salts

Directions:

1. Mix together all ingredients, making sure that they are combined well before

81

storing in an airtight container. You can use anything from a ¼ cup to a ½ cup when in severe pain in each bath.

Chapter 6. Essential Oil Blends to Use for Relief

You'll find that essential oils are great if you use them on your own, but when you put them into a blend, the effects are even better. They give you almost instant pain relief, and the right blend will target different causes and areas of your pain so that you experience overall relief. Essential oil blends should be blended in a ten millimeter rollerball bottle, and you'll want to top off with your carrier oil.

In the essential oil blends below, the carrier oil used is sweet almond oil. However, many people will use a mixture of coconut oil and sweet almond, as it's great for your skin. Apply the essential oil mixture to the affected area at the start of pain for the best results.

Essential Oil Blend #1 Calming Pain Relief

Valor essential oil is known to help calm your emotions, and lavender is meant to relieve stress. Peppermint soothes the area, and it'll help your muscles to become less stiff and tense. When added together, you can say goodbye to pain. Valor essential oil is also known to help with joint pain at the same time it helps with your muscle pain. It's commonly used for back pain.

Ingredients:

1. 10 Drops Valor Essential Oil

2. 10 Drops Lavender Essential Oil

3. 5 Drops Peppermint Essential Oil

4. Sweet Almond Oil

Directions:

1. Mix all ingredients together, and top with the sweet almond oil. Shake well before using.

Essential Oil Blend #2 Earthy Pain Relief

This is an essential oil blend with an earthy scent that will stop your back from spasming, keeping chronic pain at bay. Clary sage is known to help with inflammation as well, while the thyme essential oil will help with both joints and muscle. Rosemary helps to relax you, and it can even help to relieve headaches.

Ingredients:

1. 10 Drops Rosemary Essential Oil

2. 15 Drops Thyme Essential Oil

3. 5-8 Drops Clary Sage Essential Oil

4. Sweet Almond Oil

Directions:

1. You'll want to mix all essential oils together before adding the sweet almond oil to top it off. Remember to shake before using.

Essential Oil Blend #3 Basic Back Pain Remedy

This isn't an essential oil blend if you're suffering from chronic back pain or acute back pain. You'll find the lavender helps to relive any anxiety and stress that could be attributing to your back pain. The ginger will decrease any inflammation, and it's even known to help with joints. The peppermint will relax your muscles while improving your mood. It provides instant relief to mild back pain.

Ingredients:

1. 20 Drops Lavender Essential Oil

2. 8 Drops Ginger Essential Oil

3. 10 Drops Peppermint Essential Oil

4. Sweet Almond Oil

Directions:

1. All essential oils can be added together in
   your rollerball bottle, and then top it with
   sweet almond oil. Shake before each use.

Essential Oil Blend #5 Numbing & Powerful Relief

Clove essential oil is commonly used for tooth
pain because of its numbing effects, but it can be

used in a back pain essential oil blend as well. Yarrow is very helpful in increasing the effectiveness of this blend, as it has power anti-inflammatory effects and is known as a restorative. When combined with the roman chamomile, you'll find that this blend help with even chronic back pain. It'll even help to keep spasming from occurring and furthering the pain.

Ingredients:

1. 10 Drops Clove Essential Oil

2. 8 Drops Yarrow Essential Oil

3. 10 Drops Roman Chamomile Essential Oil

4. Sweet Almond Oil

Directions:

1. Mix all essential oils together until blended, and then top off the rest of the rollerball bottle with sweet almond oil. Make sure that you shake before applying.

Essential Oil Blend #6 Muscle Back Pain Remedy

You already know that sandalwood and wintergreen are known to help with back pain. The sandalwood will keep your tense muscles from spasming while relaxing them while the wintergreen works as an overall pain relief. White fir is what gives this essential oil blend a wood like smell, and it gets rid of those aches in your back.

Ingredients:

1. 6 Drops Sandalwood Essential Oil

2. 10 Drops Wintergreen Essential Oil

3. 15 Drops White Fir Essential Oil

4. Sweet Almond Oil

Directions:

1. All essential oils can be mixed together before finishing the bottle off with sweet almond oil. Shake well before you apply.

Essential Oil Blend #7 Nerve Pain Remedy

Chronic back pain is commonly due to nerve pain, and juniper will help with your nerve pain drastically. When paired with the vetiver essential oil in this blend, then you'll be able to relieve your general aches and pains as well as targeting your nerves. If your pain is serve, you can add up to twenty drops of the juniper essential oil to this back pain relieving blend.

Ingredients:

1. 15 Drops Vetiver Essential Oil

2. 15 Drops Juniper Essential Oil

3. Sweet Almond Oil

Directions:

1. Both essential oils can be mixed together
   and placed in the rollerball bottle. Then

top with the sweet almond oil, and shake before applying.

Essential Oil Blend #8 Mood & Muscle Relief

The lemon essential oil won't help with your back pain, but it will help with your mood and your stress, which will help to keep back pain from reoccurring. The sweet marjoram is an essential oil that will help to target the muscle pain you're feeling, while the lavender helps with anxiety and relaxes any tension.

Ingredients:

1. 10 Drops Sweet Marjoram Essential Oil

2. 5 Drops Lemon Essential Oil

3. 15 Drops Lavender Essential Oil

4. Sweet Almond Oil

Directions:

1. Mix your lavender, lemon, and sweet marjoram essential oil together in the rollerball bottle before topping it with

sweet almond oil. Shake before you apply it to the area in pain.

Essential Oil Blend #9 Stress & Inflammation Relief

This back pain essential oil blend will help by uniting the sandalwood essential oil which is known to help with stress and spasming to the frankincense which helps with inflammation. Frankincense essential oil is a powerful anti-inflammatory, and it also acts as a mild sedative, which in turn will relax you as well. The vetiver essential oil tops it off so it can help with general aches and pains.

Ingredients:

1. 8 Drops Sandalwood Essential Oil

2. 20 Drops Frankincense Essential Oil

3. 4 Drops Vetiver Essential Oil

4. Sweet Almond Oil

Directions:

1. Mix all three essential oils together, placing in the rollerball bottle before topping with sweet almond oil. Apply as needed, but shake well before each use.

Essential Oil Blend #10 Lower Back Pain Relief

Spruce is the new edition to this essential oil blend, and it's paired with something to help with spasming and general pain. The spruce essential oil adds to the blend by targeting lower back pain specifically as well as arthritis and general joint pain. It can even calm your mind and put your emotions into perspective.

Ingredients:

1. 15 Drops Spruce Essential Oil

2. 5 Drops Sandalwood Essential Oil

3. 10 Drops Lemongrass Essential Oil

4. Sweet Almond Oil

Directions:

1. All essential oils can be put into the rollerball bottle after being mixed together. Add in the sweet almond oil as your carrier oil to top it off, and shake before applying it to the area.

Essential Oil Blend #11 Strengthened Pain Relief

Copaiba helps with swelling, but it also has the added benefit of strengthening the effects of the essential oils that it's added to. It helps to boost the soothing effects of peppermint, and it helps with the general pain relief of wintergreen. This essential oil blend has a fresh, minty smell to it.

Ingredients:

1. 10 Drops Peppermint Essential Oil

2. 5-8 Drops Copaiba Essential Oil

3. 10 Drops Wintergreen Essential Oil

4. Sweet Almond Oil

Directions:

1. Mix all essential oils together before placing in the rollerball bottle.

2. Top with sweet almond oil, and shake well before applying it to the area as needed.

Chapter 7.
Supplements to Add in for Chronic Pain

You can also have various supplements that you can add into your diet if you want another natural alternative to taking care of your back pain. Many of these supplements are safe to use on a regular basis, but remember to task your doctor before adding any supplement to your daily routine. Like all medication, even natural and herbal supplements can still interact with prescription drugs and over the counter medication as well as medical conditions. Talking to your doctor before starting one is always recommended.

Supplement #1 Vitamin D

If you lack vitamin D, it can affect a lot of aspects of your health, including causing chronic back pain. If you already have back pain, a lack of vitamin D would cause it to become worse. Many conditions that have lower back pain as a symptom are resulting from vitamin D, and your doctor can recommend a dosage that is right for you. It's safe to take vitamin D as a daily supplement.

Supplement #2 Devil's Claw

Devil's claw is a wonderful herbal supplement that you can add into your diet to help reduce chronic back pain. It can even reduce flare-ups of chronic back pain. It's an African plant, and usually the daily dosage is fifty milligrams per day. It will decrease inflammation and swelling. To make sure that you have a quality supplement, look for harpagoside to be among the active ingredients of your bottle of Devil's claw.

Supplement #3 Turmeric

Turmeric is a spice that you can commonly find in your kitchen cabinet, but you'll find that it is much more effective when taken as a supplement. However, many people prefer to take it in tea or as a liquid extract. However, you cannot use turmeric powder long term, but your doctor can determine how long it is safe for you to use turmeric powder for your back pain. Prolonged use can cause stomach pain and upset. If you have a gallbladder disease, turmeric powder is not recommended. It decreased inflammation, as it is a strong anti-inflammatory, which in turn will lessen your back pain.

Supplement #4 Capsaicin

Capsaicin is the agent which gives spice to hot peppers, and it is useful when treating back pain. It helps to desensitize the channels that actually sends the pain signals to your brain's receptors, helping to decrease the pain you feel. Many people will use it in a cream, but many people believe it is more effective in treating chronic pain when taken in its supplement form.

Supplement #5 Omega-3 Fatty Acids

It's easy to find omega-3 fatty acids, and you'll find that it's easy to add into your diet. It's also meant to help reduce inflammation which is what usually causes chronic back pain, especially lower back pain. You would need to talk to your doctor about the proper dosage to help with your back pain, as it can interfere with prescription medication, such as blood thinners.

Supplement #6 White Willow Bark

Sometimes the tea doesn't work well enough, and you'll find that a white willow bark supplement can work a little better for some people. It has pain relieving properties that are similar to aspirin, but it has a much lesser risk of side effects. It is usually safe to take the pill to three times daily along with aspirin, but always talk to your doctor before adding it to your daily routine.

Supplement #7 Bromelain

You'll find that bromelain occurs naturally as an enzyme in pineapple, and it can reduce inflammation and back pain. It doesn't matter what your back pain was caused from. It can help with arthritis and joint pain as well. It's usually recommended that you take five hundred milligrams three times daily, and it's best to take it in between meals so that it is absorbed properly.

Supplement #8 Boswellia

You'll find that this is an Ayervedic herbal remedy, and it's been used for years in India. It has strong anti-inflammatory properties that are known to help with back pain, and it can usually be taken three times daily. However, you have to take it with food if you want to minimize the risk of your stomach becoming upset. Make sure each pill you're taking contains 150 milligrams of boswellic acids.

Remember:

Remember that you need to talk to your doctor before adding any supplements to your routine to treat back pain. However, you can also talk to your doctor about taking multiple supplements to help. Your doctor can talk to you about the safety precautions needed and the risks that are related to taking multiple supplements and how long you can take them safely.

Chapter 8. Extra Tips for Back Pain Relief

There are still many things that you can do to help you prevent and treat your back pain. You don't always have to use supplements or teas to help you with back pain, and instead you'll find that there are many lifestyle changes that you can make to help with your pain as well. Even chronic pain flare ups can be avoided through proper changes and tips. These bonus tips will help you to keep your back pain under control or prevent it entirely. You can even add these tips and lifestyle choices to your any natural or herbal remedies that you may already be using.

Tip #1 Make Sure Your Posture is Good

Your posture can severely effect if you have back pain or even if you suffer from chronic back pain flare ups. If you can correct your posture, then you're less likely to experience flare ups, and it'll even help to strengthen your back muscles in the process. Try to sit in chairs that help to support your back, as it'll help to encourage better posture while sitting and standing.

Tip #2 Exercise Regularly

There are two ways that exercise can help you to decrease back pain. Exercise will help you to maintain a healthy weight so that your back isn't stressed by weight it can't handle, and exercise will also help to strengthen your back muscles. Both of these factors will greatly contribute to decreasing the severity of your back pain if not solving it entirely. Exercising at least once a day for thirty minutes will make a world of difference in the pain that you're experiencing.

Tip #3 Sleep Properly

Getting enough sleep will help to reduce back pain, even chronic back pain. Your body releases tension when you get quality sleep, which keeps your muscles from overexerting themselves, and it can even ease inflammation. Make sure you have a mattress that supports your back properly so that it isn't hurting you while you sleep. Remember that soft mattresses aren't good for your back, as they push it out of alignment. A medium to firm mattress has been proven to help with back pain much more, as your back can lay naturally in any position you choose while sleeping.

Tip #4 Use Meditation

It may seem like meditation won't help on the surface, but it actually can because it helps you to relax and center yourself. This means that you'll be relaxing your muscles as well. When your mind is at rest, you'll find that your back and general muscles will start to relax. Meditating for thirty minutes each day, even if you only use deep breathing meditation, will help to keep back pain and flare-ups at bay.

Tip #5 Yoga

Yoga is also great for back pain, as it helps to increase your flexibility. Putting strain on your back is what often causes back pain, at least short term. It can even cause inflammation. When practicing yoga, you increase your flexibility, which will help you to not strain your back when going about normal activities. It also helps you to remove stress and tension from your body and mind. Practicing yoga for thirty minutes to one hour every day can make a large difference, and it's even known to help you with weight loss. Many people prefer to practice yoga in the morning, as it can help you to prepare for the day and leave any tension or stress behind.

Tip #6 Just Stretch

Sometimes the best thing to do to help decrease your chance of back pain is to stretch regularly. Touch your goes, practice various stretches, and work them into your daily routine. If you exercise daily, you can use these stretches as either a warm up or cool down before you start your daily routine. They can also help to relax you before bed. Stretches may be hard at first if you aren't flexible, but they become easier with time and practice.

It's a Process:

Remember that back pain relief won't come overnight, especially if you suffer from chronic back pain. Often, natural remedies will provide temporary relief, but with supplements and proper lifestyle changes, then you'll find you can find long term relief. Talking to your doctor and finding the right natural remedy for you and your back pain will decrease your pain and help you to live healthier and happier. Of course, it will still take time. Be patient, and combining natural remedies and solutions usually provides the best relief.

www.ingramcontent.com/pod-product-compliance
Lightning Source LLC
Chambersburg PA
CBHW071233020426
42333CB00015B/1446